Natural Remedies To Relieve Hemorrhoids

By

Gene Ashburner

ISBN-13:978-1502788443
ISBN-10:1502788446

Content

What Are Hemorrhoids?

Having hemorrhoids means that a person has a condition in which the veins around the anus or lower rectum are swollen and inflamed.

Hemorrhoids are either inside the anus or under the skin around the anus. This means that they are can be internal or external.

Many of these hemorrhoid problems will mean that any person with them will have pain or itching in that area. Hemorrhoids are usually not dangerous or life threatening.

In most cases, the symptoms will go away in a few days. Although many people with them will not experience any symptoms at all. The most common symptom of internal hemorrhoids is bright red blood covering the stool, on toilet paper, or in the toilet itself.

An internal hemorrhoid may protrude through the anus outside the body and this is what will become painful. This is called non other than a protruding hemorrhoid. This will also include swelling or a hard surface around the anus that results when a blood clot forms.

It is normal to have a hemorrhoid problem. They are very common in both men and women. Many pregnant women have to deal with the pain of hemorrhoids along with everything else that they have to go through while pregnant. Others will have hemorrhoids by the age of fifty.

In extreme cases, it may be determined by a doctor that a person must have surgery to remove the hemorrhoids.

External Hemorrhoids

Seen outside the anal opening and is covered by skin.

Black or brown in colour.

It is very painful due to the rich nerve supply in this area.

Internal Hemorrhoids

It is inside the anal canal and internal to the anal orifice.

Covered by mucous membrane and is red or purple in colour.

These hemorrhoids are painless.

Some times internal and external hemorrhoids occur in same individual.

Symptoms

Minor Hemorrhoids (internal or external) will not be painful and may go away without treatment of any kind.

A more serious hemorrhoid may bleed and you may notice blood in the toilet bowl, on the feces, on the toilet paper or on your undergarment.

If an internal hemorrhoid becomes large enough it will protrude through the anal opening. Often it can be pushed back inside if it does not go back inside by itself. These protruding internal hemorrhoids quickly become irritated and painful if they are allowed to remain outside.

External hemorrhoids can be painful when attempting to clean the anal area after a bowel movement. They are also subject to blood clots. If a blood clot forms then a painful lump may develop and the skin around the anal area will become red. This is not life threatening but it does call for medical intervention.

Pain

The anal area has many nerve endings and is sensitive to pain. External hemorrhoids can cause painful flare-ups. When internal hemorrhoids are prolapsed, they are also painful. But, not all hemorrhoids will cause you any pain.

Bleeding

The color of the blood is an indicator of the location of the bleeding

Bright red is from the anal canal

Dark red is from the colon

Bleeding does not always indicate hemorrhoids. It can also be associated with more serious medical conditions such as colorectal cancer and ulcer.

Mucus or pus

Having some mucus or pus discharge is not associated with hemorrhoids.

Change in bowel habit

When you are under emotional stress, tension, trauma, or diet change, a change will occur in your bowel habit where alternating or chronic diarrhea and constipation may happen.

Change in the shape and characteristics of your stool

When your stool is colored brown or yellow and good in form, then you have a healthy stool.

But when there is a change in the shape or color of your stool, it can be a symptom of other medical conditions but not hemorrhoids.

Swelling

A person with hemorrhoids will always have the swelling symptom, but this may also mean other medical conditions like infection.

Itching

Hemorrhoids, food and medicine allergies, skin diseases, stress, etc. can cause chronic itching.

Bulges and protrusions

Prolapsed internal hemorrhoids will cause bulges in the anal canal while external hemorrhoids will have hard bulges located outside of the opening of the anal area.

Not all of these symptoms will lead to a diagnosis of hemorrhoids.

Complications Of Hemorrhoids

Infection

The infection can spread to deep veins resulting in septicaemia.

Fibrosis

Here the hemorrhoids become fibrosed with hardening of anal orifice.

Thrombosis

Here the blood inside the hemorrhoids will form clots and can obstruct blood flow.

Gangrene

Here the tissues in the hemorrhoids and nearby skin die due to lack of blood supply.

Suppuration

When the hemorrhoids suppurate it can produce abscess with discharge of pus.

Pain

Pain is common in external hemorrhoids; which will be worse while straining at stool.

Preventing Hemorrhoids

1) Eat plenty of fruits and vegetables.

2) Take fibrous food.

3) Avoid excess intake of meat, prawns, crabs etc.

4) Keep a regular timing for food.

6) Drink sufficient quantity of water.

7) Keep regularity in bowel habits.

8) Take treatment for constipation.

Any type of strain put on the anus or anal area may cause hemorrhoids. Tiny veins surrounding the rectum become inflamed and a hemorrhoid is born. By reducing the strain put on the anus, you can reduce the possibility of getting hemorrhoids.

There are a few basic things that you can do to alter your lifestyle slightly in order to reduce the risk of developing painful hemorrhoids.

Change your diet to include foods that are high in fibre

Fibrous foods create normal stools that are able pass from the body easily. Passing stool easily creates less strain on the anal muscles and therefore reduces the risk of hemorrhoids.

Some foods that are high in fibre include:

- Grains

- Foods high in bran

- Fruits

- Vegetables

If you feel that increasing the amount of fibre in your diet is difficult by just changing your diet, there are fibre products available over the counter at your local pharmacy that will soften stool. These products usually come in powder or pill form.

Increase your water intake

The rule of thumb is to drink 8 8oz glasses of water per day. Water will loosen your stools again causing less strain on the anal muscles and decreasing your risk of painful hemorrhoids.

Change your toilet habits

Do not wait until you feel like you really have to go. Putting off going to the bathroom will give your stool time to harden while waiting in your intestines to be expelled. Hard stool cause increased pushing, which in turn causes undo stress to the anus, which increases your risk of developing hemorrhoids.

Cleanliness is next to Godliness

A clean anal area decreases the chances of developing hemorrhoids. Although cleaning with toilet paper alone is fine, there are now flushable wipes on the market that will guarantee a clean anus. They are safe to flush and safe to use in your most sensitive areas.

Exercise

Everything can be prevented, by adding a little exercise to our lives.

Long periods of sitting cause strain to the anus. As we know by now strain put on the anal muscles is what causes hemorrhoids to develop.

A rule of thumb to follow is that you should stand and walk around for at least 5 minutes every hour. Why that isn't even real sweat causing exercise. That's a simple trip to the kitchen for a glass of water!

In addition to not sitting for long periods of time, exercising regularly increases blood flow through the veins. Increased blood flow through the veins will reduce pressure on the veins surrounding the anus and therefore reduce constipation.

Risk Factors

External Hemorrhoids can also form a clot and this can be very painful; this is called a thrombosed external hemorrhoids.

Certain conditions may cause internal hemorrhoids to bulge, become irritated, and bleed, including:

Trauma during childbirth

The extra weight of pregnancy

Obesity

Chronic constipation with straining

Anal intercourse

Foods To Avoid

- Chili Peppers
- Coffee
- Alcohol
- Bad Fats
- Animal products
- Red meat

Natural Cures For Hemorrhoids

Hemorrhoids can be treated with natural products and home remedies. Severe hemorrhoids can only be treated by surgery.

Below is a list of products that can be used to cure or relieve hemorrhoids

Almond Oil

How To Use It

Apply almond oil directly onto the affected area.

How Does It Help

Effective relief from the burning and itching sensation around the anus.

Almond And Geranium Oil

How To Use It

Combine the correct ratio of these two oils. Apply the oil mixture directly to the affected area.

How Does It Help

This will assist in killing the microbes and keeps the affected area cool.

Aloe Vera

How To Use It

Apply the fresh pulp aloe vera gel directly to the anus.

How Does It Help

Aloe Vera is one of the herbs with has all of the qualities needed to repair hemorrhoidal tissue and shrink hemorrhoids. It attacks and helps to relieve the symptoms of hemorrhoids without any side effects. Pain, inflammation and enlargement of the hemorrhoids can be greatly relieved.

Apple Cider Vinegar

How To Use It

Apply the apple cider vinegar directly onto the affected area.

How Does It Help

The vinegar behaves as an astringent, decreasing the actual liquids within the swollen rectal cells. The actual apple cider vinegar additionally offers the antioxidant, beta-carotene, towards the tissue, which could reduce the chance associated with an infection

Bayberry, Goldenseal Root, Myrrh And White Oak

How To Use It

Use one of these as a salve applied directly onto the affected area.

How Does It Help

These work the same as conventional hemorrhoid treatments.

Bilberry

How To Use It

Take 100 mg three times a day of bilberry.

How Does It Help

Bilberry, particularly its extract, is being advertised as effective against several conditions such as varicose veins and hemorrhoids.

Bitter Gourd Leaves Juice

How To Use It

Extract juice from fresh bitter gourd leaves and mix 15 ml with a glass of buttermilk. Drink this in the morning.

How Does It Help

The leaves of bitter gourd vines are known to increase peristalsis to help regulate the bowel movement.

Black Fungus

How To Use It

Boil 30 grams of black fungus with 20 red dates.

Consume once per day for 10 days.

How Does It Help

Black fungus is neutral in nature and tastes sweet, which is good at cooling blood and stop bleeding. Therefore, Black fungus can be used in treatments of bloody dysentery, hematochezia and hemorrhoids.

Bovine Cartilage

How To Use It

Bovine cartilage is comprised of bone and tracheal cartilage that is derived from cows and other animals. Take it in the form of a suppository a few times a day.

How Does It Help

Hemorrhoid sufferers can use bovine cartilage to soften stools.

Buckthorn Bark, Collinsonia Root, Parsley, Red Grape Vine Leaves And Stone Root

How To Use It

These are best taken orally in capsule or tea form.

How Does It Help

They reduce pain and inflammation.

Butcher's Broom

How To Use It

Make a decoction and apply topically.

How Does It Help

It works the same as Witch Hazel, but has some additional benefits such as being able to strengthen the blood vessels. It is believed to help stop hemorrhoids from reoccurring.

Cantaloupe

How To Use It

Eat fresh cantaloupes.

How Does It Help

Cantaloupes are one of the best foods you can eat. It has a good source of vitamins and minerals. It has a high beta-carotene level and has anti-clogging properties.

Camphor

How To Use It

A topical application of Camphor is also very helpful for hemorrhoids.

How Does It Help

It is used as a "counter irritant," which reduces pain and swelling by causing irritation.

Cayenne Pepper

How To Use It

Drink a glass of cayenne pepper water daily.

How Does It Help

It will relieve the swelling and inflammation of veins and blood vessels in the rectum and anus area.

Chamomile

How To Use It

Apply chamomile ointment directly to the hemorrhoids as often as needed for relief of symptoms or drink the chamomile as a tea.

Pour a cup of not-quite-boiling water over the chamomile tea bags.

Steep for three to five minutes, cool in the refrigerator.

Apply to hemorrhoids for as long as desired.

How Does It Help

Chamomile is an anti-inflammatory. It soothes irritated tissue, reducing redness and itching.

Cherries, Blackberries, Blueberries

How To Use It

Juices are good for hemorrhoids but especially dark berry juices mixed with equal parts of apple juice. Drink at least one glass of this juice mixture each day.

How Does It Help

These berries contain "anthocyanins" and "proanthocyanidins" which reduce hemorrhoidal pain and swelling by toning and strengthening the hemorrhoid veins.

Comfrey Root

How To Use It

Make comfrey root into a paste and put into a poultice. Use on affected area.

How Does It Help

Heals bleeding caused by hemorrhoids.

Cranberry Juice

How To Use It

Puree 50 ml raw cranberries

Wrap 12,5 ml of this blend in some cheesecloth

Push it up against the anus and keep it there with some tight underwear.

After an hour or so replace it with a new batch of berries and cloth.

How Does It Help

It is high in vitamins and minerals and is effective in treating hemorrhoids since it's an anti-inflammatory and helps encourage regular bowel movements. Both are essential in getting rid of hemorrhoids.

Cumin

How To Use It

Roast 5 ml black cumin seeds.

Combine it with 5 ml un-roasted black cumin seeds.

Grind the cumin seeds together.

Consume a 2,5 ml of this powder with a glass of water once per day.

How Does It Help

Cumin seeds contain numerous phyto-chemicals that are known to have antioxidant, carminative and anti-flatulent properties. The seeds are an excellent source of dietary fibre.

Cumin may increase the motility of the gastro-intestinal tract as well as increase the digestion power by increasing gastro-intestinal enzyme secretions.

Donut Cushion

How To Use It

One can sit on it with much less pressure in the coccyx region

How Does It Help

This offers enormous relief and comfort when sitting.

Elderberries

How To Use It

Use as a poultice held to the anal area.

How Does It Help

Helps reduce swelling and inflammation.

Epsom Salts

How To Use It

Add Epsom salts to bath water.

How Does It Help

Helps relieve the pain and inflammation of hemorrhoids.

Fenugreek Seeds

How To Use It

Soak one small spoon of fenugreek seeds in water for 5 to 6 hours.

Add a cup of water.

Boil the water for 5 minutes.

Add sugar or honey for taste.

Drink it 3 times daily.

OR

Fenugreek sitz baths can be made with two or three litres of fenugreek seed extract in cold water.

How Does It Help

Fenugreek has strong medicinal healing properties.

Figs

How To Use It

Soak 3-4 figs in a glass of water overnight.

Eat the figs on an empty stomach in the morning.

How Does It Help

The small seeds in this fruit helps in bowel movement and avoid constipation.

Garlic

How To Use It

Use a pestle and mortar to squeeze all the liquid out of the cloves of garlic.

Apply the garlic juice directly to the hemorrhoids.

You should begin seeing improvements in only one week.

How Does It Help

Garlic has proven to have various medicinal properties. One of these is its ability to treat hemorrhoids.

Ginger Root

How To Use It

Ginger may be taken orally.

How Does It Help

It has been used for centuries for digestive problems but also has antioxidant and anti-microbial properties to help hemorrhoids shrink

Grape Seed Extract

How To Use It

Grape seed extracts are available in supplement form.

How Does It Help

Due to their nutritional and medicinal properties grapes, their seeds, and leaves have been used in many home remedies for centuries. Grape Seed Oil is a great source of polyphenols – flavonoids, Essential Fatty Acid – linoleic acid, vitamin E, and oligomeric proanthocyanidin.

Grape Seed Oil

How To Use It

Apply directly to affected area.

How Does It Help

It is also an excellent treatment for bleeding hemorrhoids. Grape seed oil is known to be high in essential vitamins that can strengthen the stomach and improve the body's immunity. Additionally, grape seed oil is effective for treating bleeding hemorrhoids as it can reduce bleeding. Some researches have found that grape seed oil contain natural steroids such as campesterol, beta-sitosterol and stigmasterol. This works like the topical steroid cream over the counter but without the side effects.

Horse Chestnut

How To Use It

Apply the horse chestnut ointment to affected areas.

How Does It Help

The seeds have a cooling effect on the hemorrhoid affected region and the elasticity of the veins.

Ice

How To Use It

Apply ice packs or cold compresses to your anus several times a day.

How Does It Help

It helps relieve the swelling.

Japanese Pagoda Tree

How To Use It

Even though the Japanese pagoda tree is an excellent source for an herbal hemorrhoids treatment, professionals must prepare it as improper preparation can result in a potentially poisonous concoction.

How Does It Help

The extract is used to strengthen the veins.

Key Lime

How To Use It

Take 2 pieces of the key lime tree root.

Clean it well.

Boil water (about 1 1/2 litres).

Keep the water boiling until only 1 litre remains.

Pass the water through a sieve in order to remove the root bits.

Drink the concoction every evening.

How Does It Help

It will shrink the hemorrhoids.

Lavender And Juniper Oils

How To Use It

Add 20 drops each of lavender and juniper essential oils to a hot, shallow bath, mixing the bathwater with your hand to make sure the oils are well dispersed. Soak for ten minutes.

How Does It Help

It provides relief against pain that is caused by the swollen veins in your rectum

Leeks

How To Use It

Use leeks in your cooking.

How Does It Help

Leeks can promote the circulation of Qi and scatter blood stasis in Chinese medicine.

In modern science the view is that leeks contain tough crude fibre, which is difficult for gastrointestinal digestion and absorption.

Thus leeks can increase stool bulk and promote bowel movements and prevent constipation.

Mango Seeds

How To Use It

Collect mango seeds, dry them in the shade, grind them into a powder and keep the powder in an airtight container.

This powder should be given in doses of about one and a half to two grams with or without honey as suitable two times daily

How Does It Help

Will stop the release of blood in the stools and gives relief against painful stool discharge.

Mullein

How To Use It

Make a mullein poultice and hold it to the anal area.

How Does It Help

It helps reduce swelling and inflammation.

Natto Extract

How To Use It

Natto extract is available in supplement form.

How Does It Help

Nattokinase is an enzyme derived from boiled soybeans and natto bacteria. Since painful swollen bleeding hemorrhoids are usually caused by a blood clot, Nattokinase enhances the body's natural ability to fight blood clots. It has an advantage over blood thinners because it has no reported side effects. Nattokinase prevents blood clots from forming and dissolves existing blood clots quickly, thus relieving pain and discomfort.

Neem Oil

How To Use It

Once you have cleaned your rectum and anus, apply 2 drops of neem oil to each hemorrhoid.

How Does It Help

The oil has the ability to reduce inflammation of the veins that are causing the hemorrhoids. Neem oil is also effective in reducing the pain and discomfort associated with hemorrhoids.

Oat Straw

How To Use It

Make tea from leaves

Boil the leaves and stems over a low heat for about 20 minutes.

Make tea from extract

Use 2 to 3 teaspoonfuls to one cup of boiled water and leave for about 10 minutes.

Take Tincture

Take oat straw tincture - 3 to 5 ml three times a day.

Bath

Oat straw can also be placed in a bath to soothe the skin and calm the nerves. Make an infusion with one pound of oat straw to two quarts of boiling water.

Steep in boiling water, cool a bit, and then add the brew to your bath.

How Does It Help

Oat straw and the grain are mildly antidepressant; they help in raising energy levels and support over-stressed digestive system.

Onion

How To Use It

You can take raw onion or onion juice.

If you need then you can mix some sugar or other sweetener in that onion juice.

Drink the juice.

How Does It Help

It stops the blood flow in the passage of stool.

Oranges And Bananas

How To Use It

Eat 2 to 3 oranges and 2 bananas a day.

Steam two not quite ripe bananas with their peel until they are soft.

Eat two in the morning and two in the evening.

How Does It Help

Oranges provide vitamin C, bioflavonoids, and fibre.

Bananas provide minerals that help to strengthen tissue and have plenty of fibre.

Pang Da Hai

How To Use It

It needs to be consumed as a tea on a daily basis.

How Does It Help

Promotes the movement of the intestine and create a mild laxative effect.

Papaya

How To Use It

Eat as a fruit.

How Does It Help

Papaya is an excellent fruit to eat. It has good mineral content, fibre, and has enzymes to digest protein.

Persimmon

How To Use It

Dried and frozen persimmons can be used to treat bleeding hemorrhoids, anal fissures and dry stools. They can be eaten after each meal.

How Does It Help

Dried persimmon is of cold nature and taste sweet and astringent. Dried persimmon can be used to clear heat, moisten lung, restrain intestine to stop diarrhea and bleeding, particularly for those suffer from hemorrhoids bleeding.

Petroleum Jelly Or Zinc Oxide Paste

How To Use It

Dab a small amount of Petroleum Jelly or Zinc Oxide on a cotton ball and apply to the swollen area.

How Does It Help

Petroleum Jelly and / or Zinc Oxide work as well as other expensive creams. To reduce the pain and swelling of hemorrhoids either or both can be used.

Pilewort

How To Use It

This can be used as a tincture to be directly applied to external hemorrhoids or can even be made into tea.

How Does It Help

It contains a high level of vitamin C and is said to cure hemorrhoids.

Plantain

How To Use It

Use as a poultice. It can be pounded and mashed to stop external bleeding.

OR

Plantains can be stewed, mashed, grilled, fried or boiled.

How Does It Help

This herb contains allantoin, the same soothing compound found in comfrey. It has strong anti-inflammatory properties.

Pomegranate Juice

How To Use It

Saturate a cotton ball with pomegranate juice and push it slightly into your rectum.

You can also drink the juice. It is slightly tart but is easy to drink. However, drinking more than a glass full at a time will give you an upset stomach.

How Does It Help

It is useful in reducing hemorrhoids, because of its strong astringency.

Potato

How To Use It

Small cone shaped pieces of potato used as a suppository a few times a week are also common home cures for hemorrhoids.

OR

To make a potato poultice, grate one to two tablespoons of raw potato into cheesecloth. Chill the cheesecloth and apply it to the rectal area for ten to fifteen minutes. Do this up to 3 times a day.

How Does It Help

It has a potential anti-inflammatory effect.

Pressure Relieving Exercises

How To Use It

You can also do anal exercises in your free time by simply moving your buttocks muscles around.

Hemorrhoid pillows can do the same thing if you want some additional help for your problem.

Take short walks every couple of hours just to redistribute the pressure in your anus.

How Does It Help

Hemorrhoids are the result of a pressure built up in the anal canal. There are many reasons for this mostly it is as a result of sitting or standing for too long.

Purslane

How To Use It

Use topically as a poultice.

How Does It Help

Purslane has been used throughout history in treatment of cardiac weakness, dry cough, diarrhea, dysentery, fever, gingivitis, and high cholesterol, hypertension, sore throat and urinary tract infections.

Red And Black Currant Berries

How To Use It

Drink 1 to 2 glasses of red or black currant berry juice per day

How Does It Help

Currants are high in vitamin C, rutin, and minerals. This makes their juice valuable in clearing hemorrhoids. They also have a small amount of the fatty acid GLA, which produces prostaglandin that controls body pain.

Red and black currant juice is also good for cleansing the liver and blood. Good liver function is necessary for maintaining a healthy colon, rectum and anus.

Red Sage (Salvia Officinalis)

How To Use It

In addition to red sage, you can use Vitamin E. This helps to protect against rectal damage. Take in supplement form.

How Does It Help

This herb is used for invigorating the circulation of blood and reducing stasis.

Clinical research proves that Red sage is effective in resisting bacteria, reducing inflammation, improving the cardiovascular system considerably, protecting the liver, inhibiting tumors, and normalizing the nervous system.

Used in traditional Chinese medicine, red sage root removes heat from the blood to relieve inflammation and promotes the enhanced circulation that helps keep you hemorrhoid-free.

Rutin

How To Use It

Rutin is a supplement used to treat hemorrhoids.

How Does It Help

Rutin (vitamin P) is used for poor blood circulation, hemorrhoids, Meniere's disease, varicose veins and skin bruising. It falls into a class of water-soluble plant pigments with antioxidant, anti-inflammatory, antiallergenic, antiviral and anticarcinogenic properties. Rutin is abundant in buckwheat, apricots, cherries, prunes and rose hips. It is a greenish/yellow, solid substance.

Sesame Seeds Decoction

How To Use It

Boil 20 g of sesame seeds in 500 ml of water.

Cook until the volume is reduced to 1/3.

Drink the decoction.

How Does It Help

They contain valuable vitamins and fibre essential for digestion and diet.

They also contain a huge amount of copper, which is known to have excellent anti-inflammatory properties.

Sitz Bath

How To Use It

Fill your bath with three to four inches of warm water.

Don't add anything to the water.

Sit in the tub for 15 minutes.

Repeat this several times a day.

OR

Pour boiling water over 2 oz rosemary, 1 oz chamomile, 1 oz chickweed, 1 oz marshmallow root, 1 oz plantain, 1 oz calendula and 2 oz sea salt.

Allow the tea to steep for 4 hours.

Strain the mixture.

Pour into a bowl and sit with the irritated area in the tea for about 15 minutes.

How Does It Help

Warm water relaxes the sphincter muscle, which can help soothe the pain associated with hemorrhoid protrusions.

Sulphur And Vaseline

How To Use It

Mix some sulphur with Vaseline and use as a salve.

How Does It Help

Effective for temporary relief from the discomfort, swelling and mild pain of hemorrhoids.

Sweet Clover

How To Use It

How Does It Help

Sweet clover is believed to help with unabridged circulatory problems, which will help get those swollen blood vessels back to a general size.

Tea Tree Oil

How To Use It

Use as an astringent directly onto the affected area.

How Does It Help

Many health benefits can be attributed to tea tree essential oil because it contains properties like anti bacterial, anti microbial, anti septic, anti viral, balsamic, cicatrisant, expectorant, fungicide, insecticide, stimulant and sudorific. So it is not surprising that it can also treat hemorrhoids.

The tea tree essential oil is actually not extracted from the common plant of tea. Instead, it is extracted through steam distillation of twigs and leaves of Tea Tree.

Tomatoes

How To Use It

Use as a poultice.

Take 1 ripe tomato and split in half.

Apply pressure in the anal sphincter. You can sit or lie on top with the tomato applied with gauze.

How Does It Help

The tomato is an ally to those suffering from hemorrhoids, and provides immediate relief.

Turnip Juice

How To Use It

Extract juice from turnip leaves.

Mix the 50 ml turnip juice, 50 ml watercress juice, 50 ml spinach juice and 50 ml carrot juice.

Drink the juice immediately.

How Does It Help

Turnips are excellent for hemorrhoids treatment but do not drink the turnip juice on it's own.

Vicks Vaporub

How To Use It

Apply directly onto affected area.

How Does It Help

Serves as an astringent to shrink the hemorrhoids.

Warm And Cold Compress

How To Use It

Put some ice into a plastic bag and place the ice bag to the inflamed area for ten minutes at a time, every couple of hours or so.

Once you are done with the cold compress, apply a hot compress to the area for further relief from pain.

How Does It Help

Warm and cold compress are known to be a great hemorrhoids remedy for pain relief.

Washing Techniques

How To Use It

You must maintain a clean anus at all times if you want to avoid infection and heal as quickly as possible. To clean your anus you will need to shower often and also use mild soap in the area. You can also use baby wipes throughout the day after you pass a stool because they will have a built in cleaning solution. These will also be more soothing on your rectum. Less irritation will yield faster healing times as a result.

How Does It Help

This is one of the simplest hemorrhoid remedies to abide by, but it can make a huge difference in your healing. You must get a full night of sleep any time you can, and it would be a good idea to take naps throughout the day as well if you have the chance. A few days of bed rest may be all your body needs to get better.

White Radish And Honey

How To Use It

Grate the white radish finely in order to extract the juice it has from the plant itself. Add a bit of honey.

Apply the mixture directly onto the hemorrhoids.

Continually do this every day for 2 weeks.

How Does It Help

It will heal the hemorrhoids in a couple of days.

Witch Hazel

How To Use It

Witch hazel applied with a cotton ball a few times a day acts as astringent.

How Does It Help

It is known for its anti-inflammatory properties, its anti-oxidant properties, and especially because of its astringent properties.

Tannins produced in the witch hazel tree act on human tissue by causing it to shrink, which is just the ticket when you have hemorrhoids.

Yarrow

How To Use It

Yarrow boiled into a tea and applied with a cotton ball several times a day is another anti-inflammatory agent.

How Does It Help

It is known for its anti-inflammatory properties, its anti-oxidant properties, and especially because of its astringent properties.

Zinc Oxide Treatment

How To Use It

Apply zinc oxide cream to your rectal area with a clean cotton ball. Do not glob the cream on. Spread an even layer over the rectal area.

How Does It Help

Zinc oxide creates a barrier over the skin to protect it from irritation. Using zinc oxide on your hemorrhoids may provide relief from anal irritation and itching, which is part of the symptoms of hemorrhoids.

Use Fruit Juices To Relieve Constipation

Fruit juices are an excellent way to stimulate your colon and other parts of the body. Since your colon is less active at night, drinking juices as soon as you awaken and get up can stimulate strong peristaltic action and promote a bowel movement.

Vegetables like fruits and their juices have healing properties because of the fibre, antioxidants, vitamins, and minerals they have. For constipation, vegetables are an excellent source of minerals and fibre. In addition there are specific vegetables and their juices that stimulate the colon become more active.

Juices are absorbed quickly into your bloodstream. As a result, your cells are provided quickly with nutrients that feed them and that wash away waste. Juices give you the opportunity to get quick relief from various body conditions such as constipation. Juices move into your colon quickly to cleanse it and to activate peristaltic action.

Eating and drinking vegetables and their juices provide you with minerals and nutrients that build your blood, tissue, bones, and cells. It is minerals that build every part of your body. It is minerals that keep your body's pH at the required level. It is minerals that keep your body alkaline by neutralizing body acids.

It is minerals that build your colon wall tissues and cells so your colon can perform those activities that prevent constipation.

Apples And Apple Juice

Apples are good for eliminating constipation because they are high in pectin, a soluble fibre, have many minerals, and contain sorbitol - a natural sugar, which stimulates peristaltic action. Pectin helps to detoxify the intestines and promote regular bowel movements.

The fibre in apples adds weight and bulk to your fecal matter and helps draw water from your colon into the fecal matter keeping the stool from becoming hard and thus preventing constipation.

Apples are one of best fruits to eat because they are high in minerals, which provide alkaline electrolytes to your body. What electrolytes do is neutralize acids that are created during illness, anxiety, anger, exercising, breathing pollution, and improper eating. Body acid is a major reason we get deadly diseases as we age

Make eating apples or drinking fresh apple juice a daily habit. They are also effective in liver and gallbladder problems.

Here's what to do

Use crisp and hard apples such as granny smith, Fuji, or gala apples for juicing.

Drink 3 glasses of apple juice during the day - morning, noon, and evening.

In combination with drinking fresh apple juice, eat 3 to 4 apples each day to get fibre. The combination of eating and drinking apples juice will activate your colon to start moving stagnant matter.

One Day Apple And Apple Juice Fast

You can also do a 1 day or 2 day apple and apple juice fast.

Eat 3 to 4 apples during the day.

Drink apple juice every 2 hours.

Don't eat anything until the next morning. Then, start changing your eating habits.

Apple And Pear Juice

Prepare equal amounts of fresh apple and pear juice.

Drink this combination when you first wake up and one hour before bedtime.

Juice the pears that are slightly hard. If the pear is ripe, it is best to blend it whole with apple juice to create a thick drink. Using the whole pear will give you additional fibre. Just remove the seeds but do not peel organic pears.

Pears have minerals, vitamins, and chemicals that help to clean out your colon, kidney and to regenerate your blood cells.

Apple Juice And Prune Juice

Drink 3 to 4 glasses of apple juice a day.

To speed up the laxative effects of apple juice, take the following combination first thing in the morning before you have breakfast:

Drink 2 to 3 cups of prune juice.

After ½ hour drink one cup of apple juice

Then 1 hour later drink another cup of apple juice.

Prune juice by itself is good for constipation. It is a safe, gentle and an effective laxative. Drink a cup in the morning and a cup in the evening. Prune juice contains the substance dihydrophenylisatin, which is responsible for the laxative action. Prunes are also high in iron and are a great supplement if you are anaemic or low on iron.

If you add prune juice to your diet, do not drink as much of it as you would when you have constipation.

Drink ½ glass in the morning and perhaps ½ glass in the evening.

Grapefruit

Another constipation remedy you can use is drinking a glass of fresh squeezed grapefruit first thing in the morning.

Again wait at least 1/2 hour before you eat anything.

If you are taking any anticonvulsant drugs, birth control pills, estrogen, protease inhibitors and even other types of drugs avoid drinking grapefruit juice. It slows the breakdown of certain drugs allowing them to increase in the blood to dangerous levels.

Lemons

Lemons are filled with minerals, especially potassium, Vitamin C, and bioflavonoids. They have a cleansing action for the entire body.

Fresh lemon juice is the king of fruit juices. It contains citric acid, which acts in the body in a way no other juice does.

First it acts on the liver to build up its enzymes so it can detoxify toxins in the blood. Then it combines with calcium to form soluble chemical substances. This makes it effective in removing kidney and pancreatic stones, plack build up along artery walls, and other calcium deposits that occur in the body.

When the liver, gallbladder, and pancreas are not working right, food digestion is affected. This in turn will create constipation.

Use lemons moderately since they break up oils during digestion and in our body they make oils less available to our cells and joints.

If you have lemon allergies or ulcers then you should avoid lemon juice. If you have arthritis lemons are not a good choice.

Here's what to do:

Squeeze one lemon into a glass of warm distilled water.

Drink it first thing when you wake up.

Don't drink anything else for at least 1/2 hour

Orange And Grapefruit Juice

Drink a combination of grapefruit and orange juice first thing in the morning. Just prepare a half and half drink of these citrus fruits.

Papaya

Papaya not only aids digestion but also helps prevent constipation. It provides relief from piles and also has anti-cancer properties. Papaya has also been shown to lower cholesterol levels, prevents the formation of urinary stones, it prevents intestinal infection by parasites and aids in the proper functioning of the body's immune system.

For lactating mothers, according to traditional beliefs, papaya also helps to stimulate milk production.

Papayas contain papain, an enzyme that helps digest proteins (especially food with gluten). Concentrated amounts can especially be found in unripe papaya. This enzyme helps prevent the accumulation of mucoprotein (partially digested protein) in the body and lymphatic system. In fact, papain has been extracted to make dietary supplements for digestion.

The unripe papaya is considered to have more healing powers for constipation than the ripe one.

Papayas are a good source of fibre. Its fibre is able to keep cancer-causing toxins in the colon away from the healthy colon cells. Those who are experiencing constipation or at risk of colon cancer should consider taking more papaya. Papaya's folate, vitamin C, vitamin A, beta-carotene and vitamin E have been linked with reduced risk of colon cancer.

Additionally, the antioxidant nutrients found in papaya have also been proven to reduce muscle inflammation and the healing of burns and wounds.

Papaya Milk Energy Drink

Cut papaya and blend with milk in a 50/50 mix

Add honey if desired.

Papaya Salad

Shred green papaya
Add sliced tomatoes.
For dressing
Chopped garlic
25 ml fish sauce
12,5 ml limejuice
Cilantro
Thai basil
5 ml chopped mint
Chili padi
Sugar to taste

Unripe Papaya Juice

Peel off skin and put in blender.

This recipe is especially good for the lymphatic system and after a meal that is heavy in gluten.

Rhubarb

Rhubarb has a strong laxative action so it is best to use it with other juices.

Here's how you can use this herb.

This tart drink will help you with your constipation.

Ingredients

> 3 stalks of rhubarb (leaves removed - don't use rhubarb leaves since they contain toxic chemicals)
> 250 ml fresh apple juice
> 1 quart peeled lemons
> 12,5 ml honey

Method

Blend together in a blender.

Drink 1 glass 3 times a day.

You may add more syrup if the taste if to harsh for you.

Use rhubarb raw since it is high in oxalic acid. Use it sparingly and do not cook it. Cooking converts the organic oxalic acid into inorganic oxalic acid. The body does not easily absorb inorganic oxalic and it forms crystal deposits in the kidney and throughout the body.

If you have arthritis or gout, do not use rhubarb.

Green Drink For Constipation

A green drink is a powerful drink that can help detoxify your colon and your blood. This drink keeps your colon and your whole body working better and longer.

Ingredients

1 to 2 oz of pure liquid chlorophyll
Juice of 1 lemon
250 ml distilled water

Method

Combine all the ingredients together.

Drink a glass of this green drink every morning.

Herbs And Seeds For Constipation

Cayenne

Cayenne is a constipation remedy that is effective in producing peristalsis in your colon and aids digestion. It can be used regularly at every meal and when needed for constipation. Cayenne pepper is known to help thin the blood. So, it is good for improving blood circulation.

Cayenne when used with other herbs helps to deliver these herbs more efficiently to where they are needed in the body.

Do not use cayenne seeds, as they can be toxic. If you are pregnant or breast-feeding do not take cayenne supplements.

Cayenne has the ability to block the ulcer producing effect of NSAIDS. It also has shown to increase the body's absorption of theopylline, a drug used to treat asthma.

One of the most effective stimulants, mostly, cayenne targets the digestive and the circulatory system. Cayenne regulates blood pressure, strengthens the pulse, feeds the heart, lowers cholesterol, and thins the blood. It cleanses the circulatory system, heals ulcers, stops haemorrhaging, speeds healing of wounds, rebuilds damaged tissue, eases congestion, aids digestion, regulates elimination, relieves arthritis and rheumatism, prevents the spread of infection and numbs pain.

Sesame Seeds

Black sesame seeds provide nutrition and action on the liver, intestines, kidney, and blood.

Grind black sesame seeds into a meal by using a small coffee grinder. Mix the ground black sesame seeds with dark honey and form into small balls. Eat one 3 times a day dipped in rice wine.

You can also prepare a sesame seeds soup with brown rice:

Ingredients

Sesame seeds
Brown rice
Distilled water

Method

Soak 10 parts of sesame seeds with 1 part brown rice in distilled water

After they are soft, about an hour, pour out the water grind them in a small food grinder to produce liquid. Strain the remaining liquid to remove coarse particles.

Dilute liquid with distilled water and add some honey.

Cook on low heat until liquid becomes syrupy

Drink around two cups to relieve constipation with in hour or so.

Sunflower Seeds

Sunflower seeds promote regularity. They contain omega-6 fatty acid just like olive oil.

Use them raw, shelled and unsalted.

Grind the seeds and add them to your morning smoothie, salad dressing or morning cereal.

Sunflower Drink

Ingredients

> 25 ml ground sunflower seeds
> 250 ml boiling water
> 10 ml honey

Method

Combine the ingredients together.

Mix well.

Drink this combination morning and night to help you with you constipation.

Brewer's Yeast

Brewer's yeast can help to ease, reduce, or clear your constipation. If you can handle the taste, add it to your juices morning and night.

Brewer's Yeast contains all B vitamins, except B12. It also contains many vitamins, minerals and is high in amino acids.

When you first use brewer's yeast, it will create gas in your colon. Brewer's yeast supplements your good bacteria in your colon, increasing its count. This increase in good bacteria activates a battle between the good and bad bacteria creating gas as a by-product. Keep using brewer's yeast until the gas stops. This may take a few weeks but you are doing one of the best things you can do for your health - increasing good bacteria and reducing bad bacteria.

You can improve the benefit of using brewer's yeast by eating cultured yoghurt or supplement good bacteria capsules between meals. You want to do this between meals so when you take your supplement your stomach does not put out to much HCl acid, which would kill the good bacteria.

If you have gout or are taking monoamine oxidase inhibitors do not take brewers yeast.

Organic Sulphur (MSM)

MSM stands for methyl sulfonyl methane. MSM is organic sulphur. It provides many benefits in the body and is widely used as an anti-inflammatory. MSM is especially good for relieving constipation.

MSM in your colon stops or blocks the activity of cholinesterase (ko-li-nes-ter-ace.)

What is cholinesterase?

Our nervous system is composed of a network of nerve cells, which start at the brain and end on all parts of our body. It is nerves that direct muscle contraction or expansion for your bowel movements. After the muscle completes its movement, an enzyme cholinesterase is released, which stops the muscle from moving again. Without the nerve signal blocking cholinesterase, the muscle would continue to move non-stop.

MSM is useful in clearing up constipation. As MSM blocks the activity of cholinesterase, it allows more peristaltic action to occur in your colon.

The action that MSM has in your colon is useful for older people who have less nerve signals for peristalsis.

A Morning Smoothie To Stop Constipation

Ingredients

1 banana (peeled)
5 strawberries
12,5 ml lecithin granules
10 ml flax seed oil
250 ml almond milk
250 ml apple juice
Brown sesame seeds (ground)
Sunflower seeds (ground)
Flax seeds (ground)
Almonds (ground)
5 ml honey (optional)

Method

Blend the ingredients together in a blender until smooth.

Why the seeds and nuts?

Brown sesame seeds - are high in lecithin, vitamin C, E, and Calcium. They improve liver function and help in constipation

Sunflower seeds - are high protein, Calcium, and iron. They are one of the best natural foods, which feed the entire body.

Flax seeds - are high in fibre and provide bulk for your stools.

Almonds - use around 6 to 7 or more. They are high in Calcium, Phosphorus and have some B-vitamins. Only eat a few. They are high in calories.

Eating Bran To Eliminate Constipation

One reason many people are constipated is they don't eat a lot of fibre. Most people only eat about 8 mg of fibre per day. To have good health and have good elimination, you need around 30- 35 mg of fibre.

Eating bran is one of the quickest and best ways to increase your fibre. It will increase the weight and size of your stools more than the fibre contained in fruits or vegetables. Bran is the outer husk of the grain - wheat, corn, rice, and oat - which is indigestible.

It does not irritate the lining of the stomach, small intestine or your colon. It is not a laxative but promotes the movement fecal matter through your colon in a natural way. Unlike drugstore laxatives or other natural strong laxatives, bran does not quickly purge out all the contents in your colon.

Use 1 or 2 heaped tablespoons of bran in your morning cereal, in your baking, and in your smoothies.

Health Alert

When using bran, make sure you drink plenty of water during the day to keep your stools soft.

Here are some other ways to use bran.

- ❖ Baked breads, muffins and other baked goods
- ❖ Breaded mixes
- ❖ Hamburger meat
- ❖ Juices
- ❖ Pancake or waffle mix
- ❖ Salads
- ❖ Scramble eggs
- ❖ Soups
- ❖ Stuffing
- ❖ Vegetarian burger mix
- ❖ Yogurt

When you put bran in juice or any liquid just eat it with a spoon.

How much bran should you take for good bowel regularity? Each person is different. You need to experiment. Start with two teaspoon each day and work towards 10 teaspoons a day or until you have bowel movements without effort or straining.

There are four basic bran products

- ❖ Wheat
- ❖ Corn
- ❖ Oats
- ❖ Rice

They all provide a solid source of fibre in varying amounts. Make sure the bran you use is 100% unprocessed bran.

Use bran for a few weeks to get your bowel movements back to normal. Eating bran should get your bowels moving in a few days or less.

Once your bowels are back to normal, back off from using a lot of bran and depend more on fibre from eating more fruits, vegetables, nuts, and seeds.

There are many new products, which use bran added to other nutrients or powders. Although these can be useful, use them for a limit time.

Constipation Remedy Using Potassium And Prunes

Potassium and prunes are a natural constipation remedy that you can quickly use to help you get constipation relief.

Potassium is needed in your colon walls to insure that peristaltic action occurs. Without potassium, colon walls are weak and unable to respond and contract properly when fecal matter needs to be move.

Potassium in your colon wall tissues brings in more oxygen, which is required for good cell function and elimination of toxins. In addition, potassium creates an alkaline environment inside and outside the cell, which help protect cell walls from bacteria, fungus, and other pathogens.

Potassium is a powerful source when it comes to cleaning, feeding and building your colon walls. Removing the thin layer of build up – harden mucus, dried fecal matter, waste derby, heavy metals - against your colon wall can be accomplished by eating those foods that are high in potassium.

Excess build up on your colon walls of fecal matter and toxins is a cause of continual constipation. This build up prevents your colon walls from functioning properly.

Potassium is necessary for reducing anxiety and depression. These conditions can affect peristaltic movements of your colon. Lack of it causes muscles and organs to sag and lack tone.

Potassium, also, draws water out of the body. So when potassium is in your colon it attracts water and pulls it into the fecal matter. This makes your fecal matter softer and easier to move along the colon.

To get more potassium into your diet make a constipation remedy drink by,

Pouring hot water over dried prunes and waiting 10 minutes. Then eat the prunes and drink the juice Do this on an empty stomach in the morning.

The high concentration of potassium and vitamin A, in prunes, stimulates enzymatic processes. These processes melt down fecal wall wastes and dissolve blockages. They also activate peristaltic action to move this waste out through your rectum.

The foods to eat that are high in potassium are:

Kale, cabbage, yellow tomatoes, spinach, carrots, broccoli, cucumbers, cauliflower, alfalfa sprouts, goat milk, sesame seeds, wheat germ brewers yeast, flax seed, grapes, green peppers, pineapple, beets, potatoes with skin Blackstrap molasses

If you have any kidney disease, do not take potassium supplements unless directed by your doctor. If you are pregnant, take potassium only under a doctor's direction.

If you are on any type of drugs, do not take potassium unless directed by your doctor.

When you have constipation it is best to take potassium supplement. Once you have your constipation eliminated back off on the potassium you are taking and depend on your potassium dose from the foods you eat.